MW01446164

CHARLIE'S ANATOMICAL ADVENTURES

THE HEART

Little Creek Press
MINERAL POINT, WISCONSIN

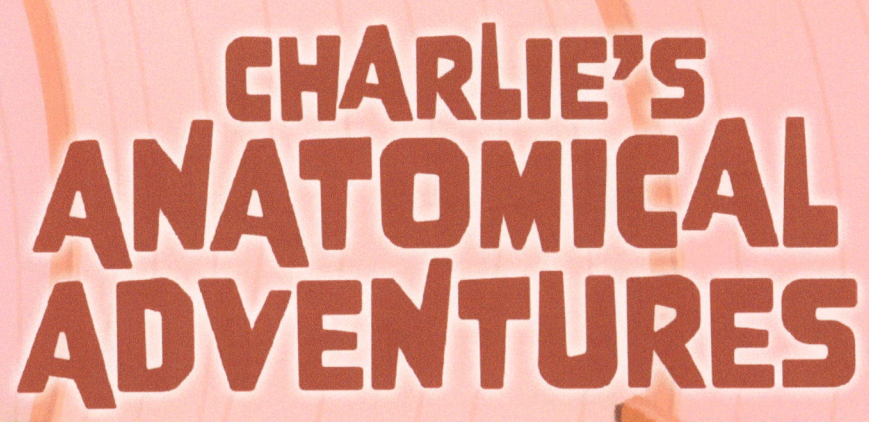

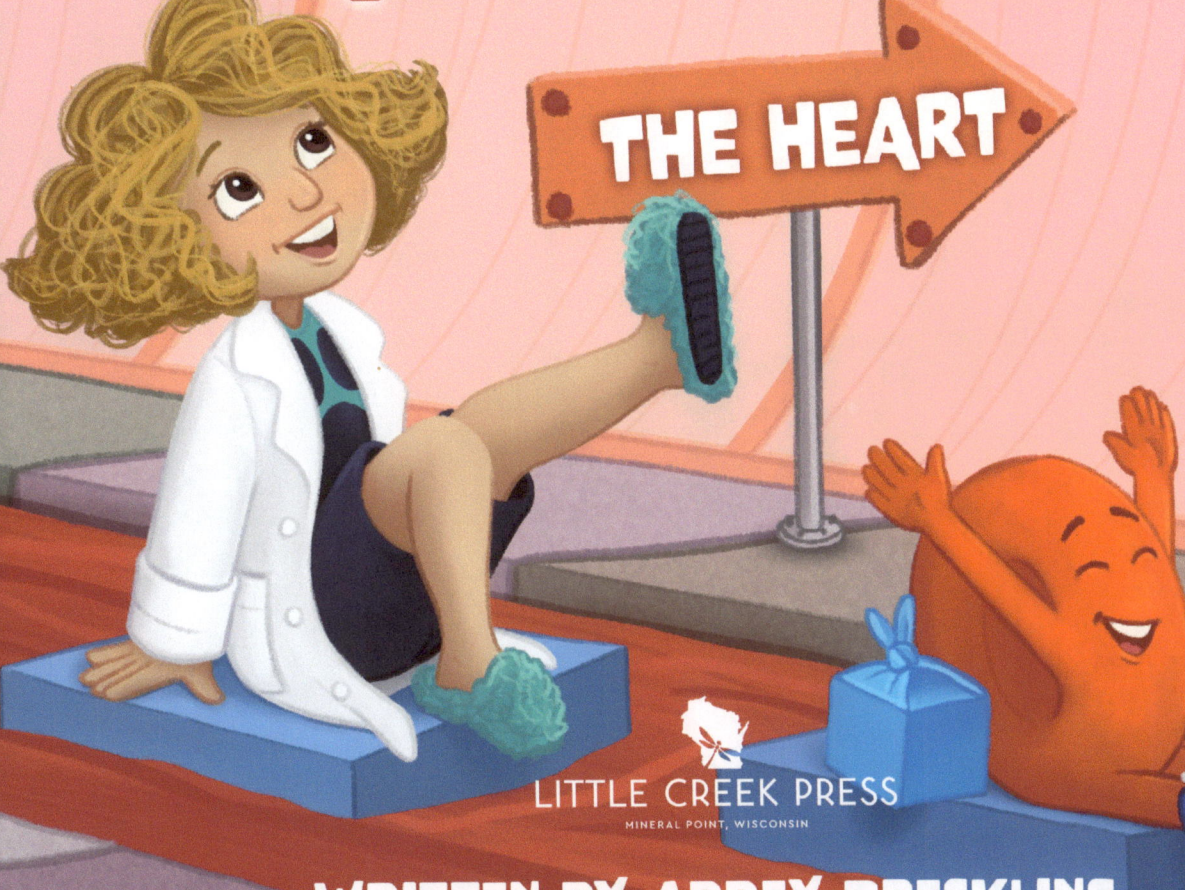

WRITTEN BY ABBEY BRECKLING
ILLUSTRATED BY MELISSA LETTIS

Copyright © 2025 Abbey Breckling
Illustrations © 2025 Melissa Lettis

All rights reserved. No part of this publication may be reproduced, distributed, or transmitted in any form or by any means, including photocopying, recording, digital scanning, or other electronic or mechanical methods, without the prior written permission of the publisher, except in the case of brief quotations embodied in critical reviews and certain other noncommercial uses permitted by copyright law. For permission requests or other information, please send correspondence to the following address:

Little Creek Press
5341 Sunny Ridge Road
Mineral Point, WI 53565

ORDERING INFORMATION
Quantity sales. Special discounts are available on quantity purchases by corporations, associations, and others. For details, contact info@littlecreekpress.com

Orders by US trade bookstores and wholesalers.
Please contact Little Creek Press or Ingram for details.

Printed in the United States of America

Cataloging-in-Publication Data
Names: Breckling, Abbey, author; Lettis, Melissa, illustrator
Title: Charlie's Anatomical Adventure: The Heart
Description: Mineral Point, WI, Little Creek Press, 2025
Identifiers: LCCN: 2024924106 | ISBN: 978-1-955656-88-7
Classification: JUVENILE NONFICTION / Concepts / Body
JUVENILE NONFICTION / Science & Nature / Anatomy & Physiology
JUVENILE NONFICTION / Health & Daily Living / Bodily Functions

Book design: Little Creek Press

From the bottom of my heart (and every chamber in between), I want to give a huge "thank you" to all the wonderful people who made this book possible! To our loving golden doodle, Charlie, who inspired the bright, curious, and adventurous spirit of this story—you are truly the heartbeat of this project.

To my amazing family and friends, thank you for pumping me full of encouragement and keeping the flow of ideas strong. Your support and input helped me by bringing this long-awaited dream to life. You've all been the oxygen to my inspiration, and this book would not have been complete without you. Thank you for making my anatomical adventure so memorable!

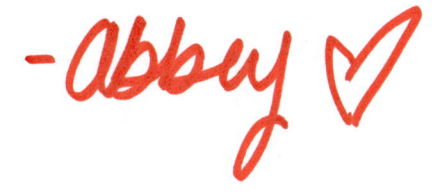

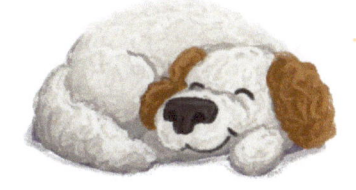

-Abbey ♡

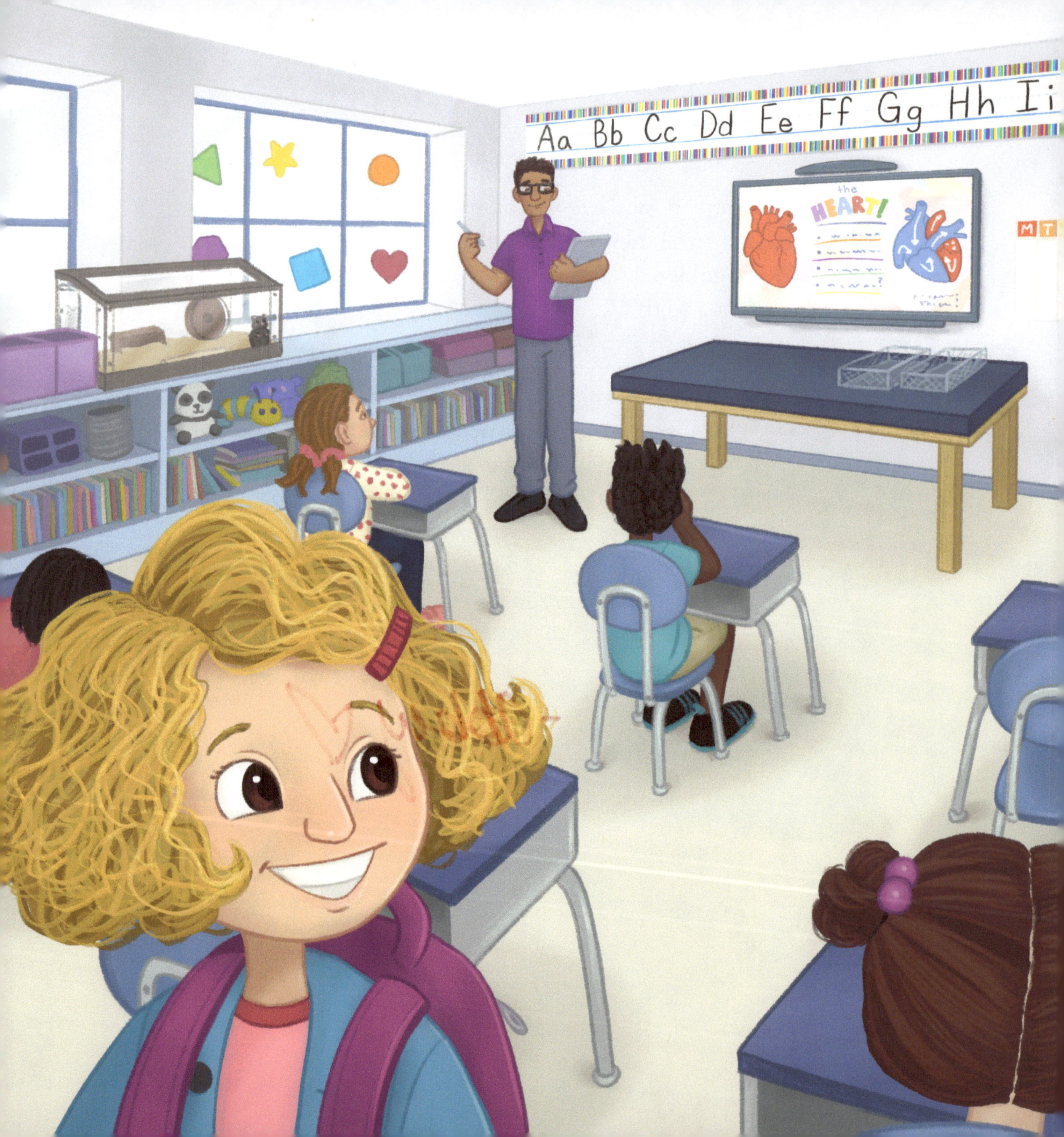
Aa Bb Cc Dd Ee Ff Gg Hh Ii
the
HEART!

In a bright, lively classroom, excitement fills the air as Charlie and her classmates are ready to explore something amazing. Today's science lesson is about the **heart**—the incredible **organ** that keeps our bodies alive!

"The **heart** has an important job," their teacher says. "It works like a pump, pushing blood all around your body including, your **brain**, **muscles**, and every single **organ**."

Charlie stands near the back of the room, her eyes sparkling with curiosity as she eagerly takes in every word. She can't wait to learn more about this fantastic part of her body!

"Does everyone's **heart** look like this?" Charlie asks, raising her hand high in the sky. "It looks like an upside-down pyramid with tubes, like spaghetti, coming out of the top!"

"Great thought, Charlie!" says their teacher, smiling. "Those tubes are called **arteries** and **veins**. Think of them as highways for your blood! **Arteries** carry blood away from the **heart** to the rest of your body, and **veins** bring blood back to the **heart**."

The students lean closer as the teacher continues. "A healthy **heart** has strong, muscular walls and a little bit of fat around it, called **adipose** tissue, which helps protect it. Inside, the **heart** has **chambers**, special spaces where blood is pumped or pushed to travel all around your body."

Charlie beams, already imagining her **heart** hard at work. "Wow, that's amazing!" she says.

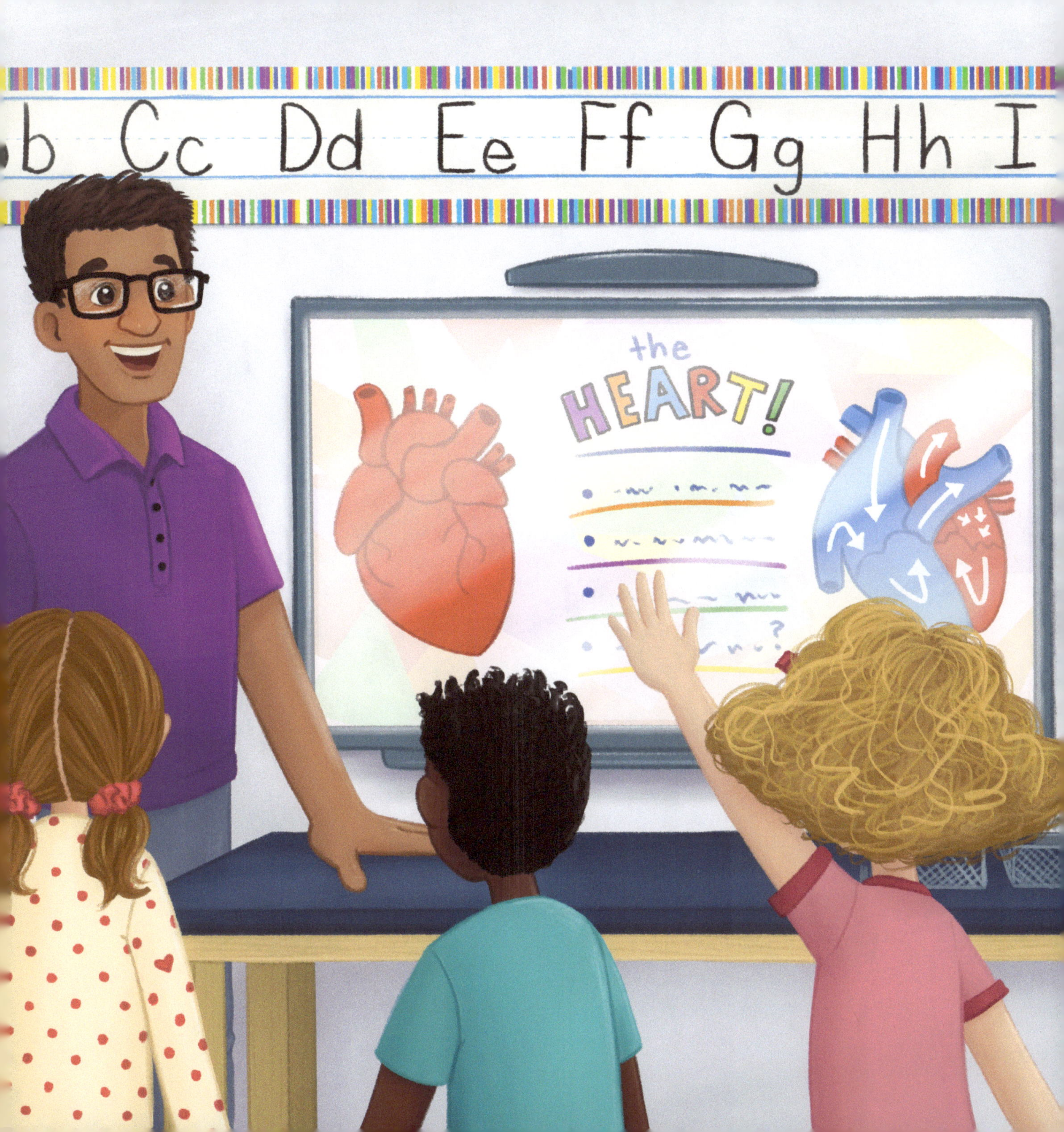
b Cc Dd Ee Ff Gg Hh I
the HEART!

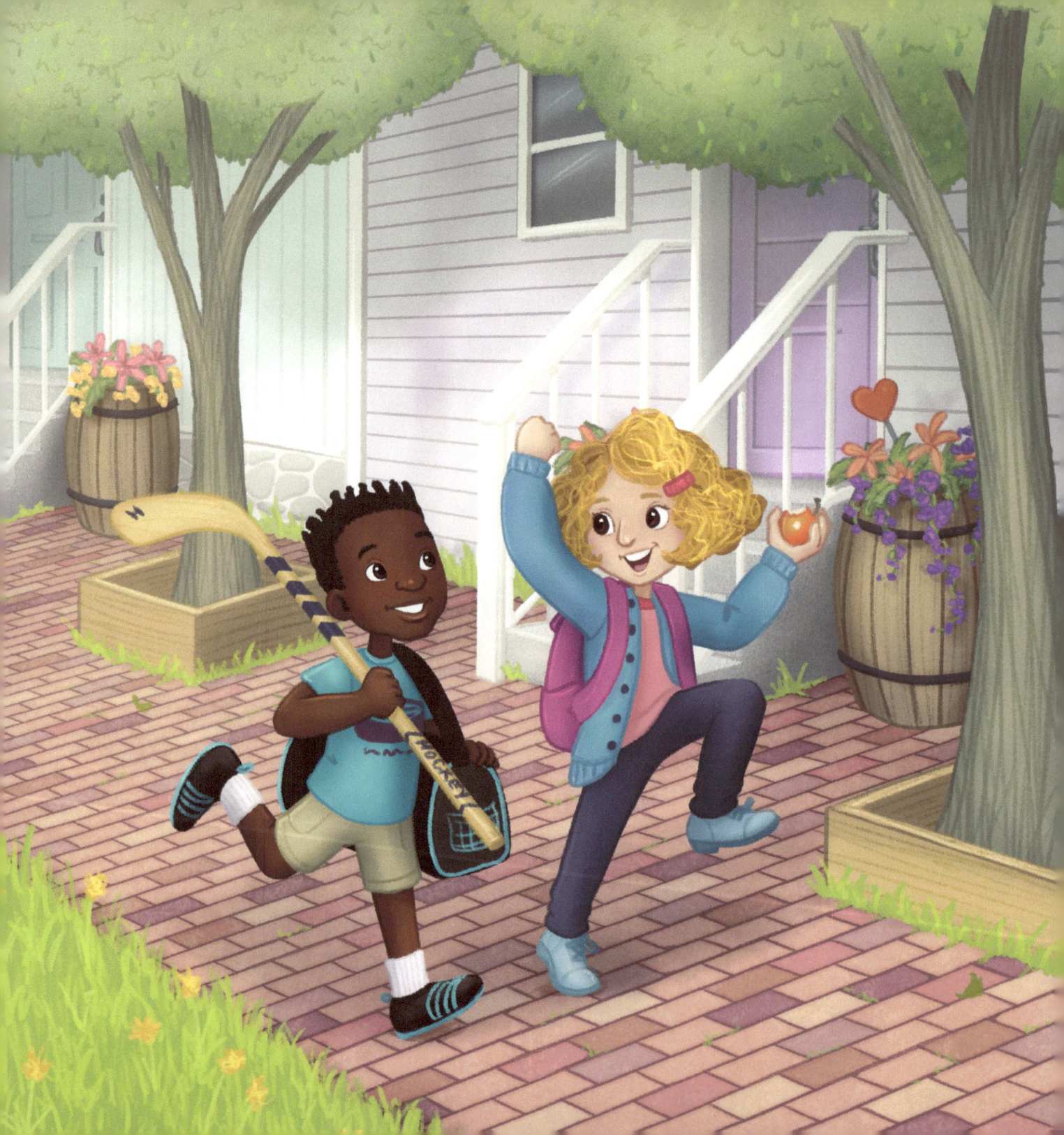

On their walk home from school, Charlie and her friend Owen can't stop talking about today's science lesson. "Did you know that regular **exercise** and eating healthy foods can help keep your **heart** strong?" Charlie says, holding up her apple with a grin.

"Yep! My mom is a **cardiologist**, and she teaches me all about the **heart**," Owen replies, balancing his hockey stick on his shoulder.

Charlie looks thoughtful. "What does my **heart** look like? If it's always pumping, even when I'm eating, running, or jumping, does that mean my **heart** is healthy? I love playing outside, so I must have a super-strong muscle pump!"

Owen laughs and nods. "I bet my **heart** beats at least 120 times a minute while playing hockey! It beats faster so my **muscles** get the **oxygen** and **nutrients** they need to keep going!"

The two friends skip happily down the sidewalk, thinking about how they can keep their **hearts** healthy and strong.

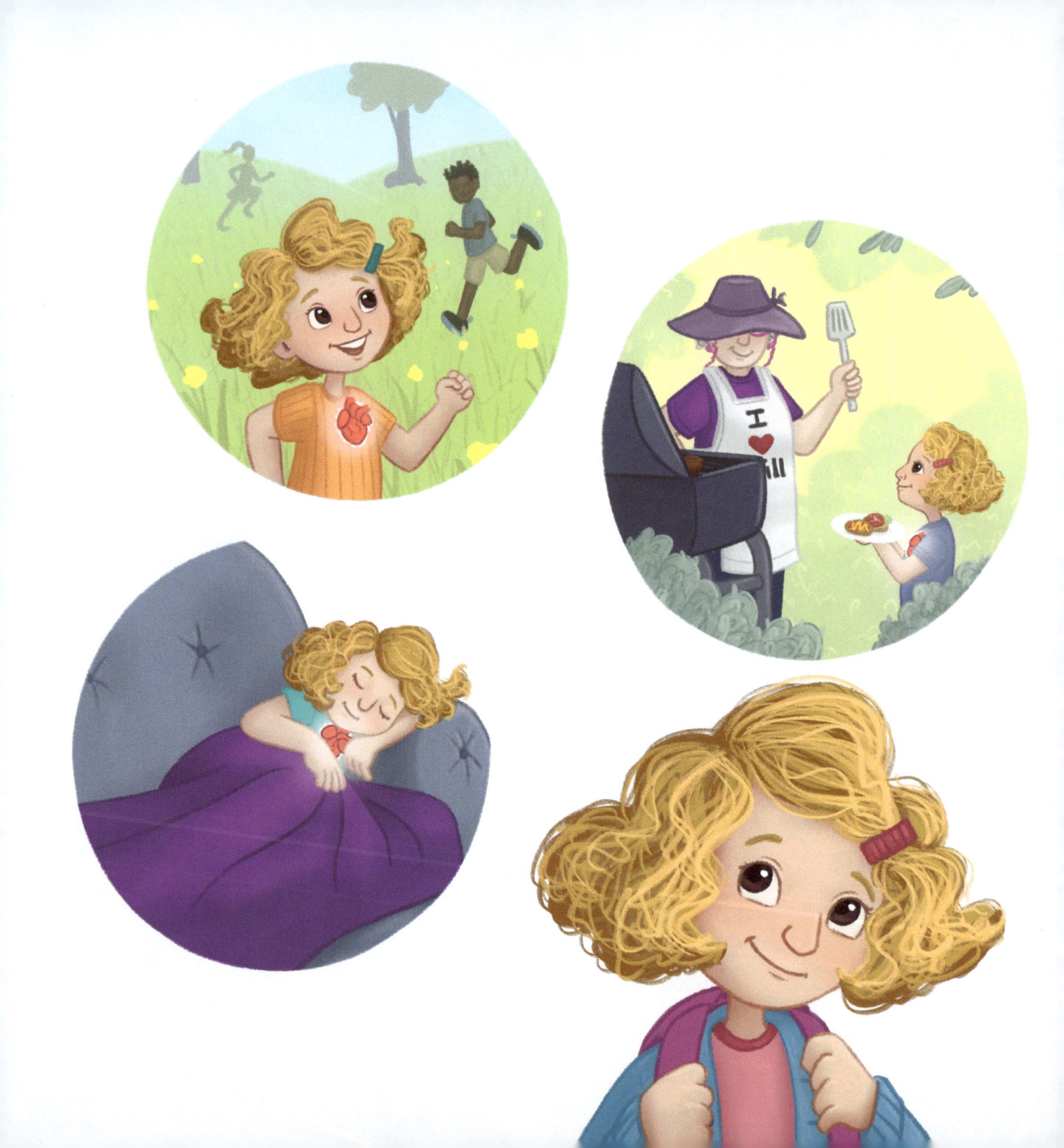

As Charlie skips home, her imagination comes alive! She pictures her **heart** as a cheerful little pump, always hard at work to keep her body and mind working.

Charlie smiles to herself and thinks, "My **heart** is amazing! It pumps blood to all my **organs** when playing tag with my friends, enjoying dinner with my family, or curling up under my blanket to rest. My **heart** keeps pumping so I can do all the things I love with my family and friends!"

Charlie bursts into the living room at home, her arms stretched wide with excitement. "Guess what I learned in school today?" she exclaims, her voice full of energy. "We talked about a super cool muscle pump in our bodies called the **heart**! It has four **chambers** that work together to squeeze blood, sending **oxygen** and **nutrients** all over our bodies, right down to our tiniest **cells**."

Her family listens carefully, smiling as Charlie shares what she learned. Her excitement fills the room, making everyone eager to hear more about the incredible **organ**, the **heart**!

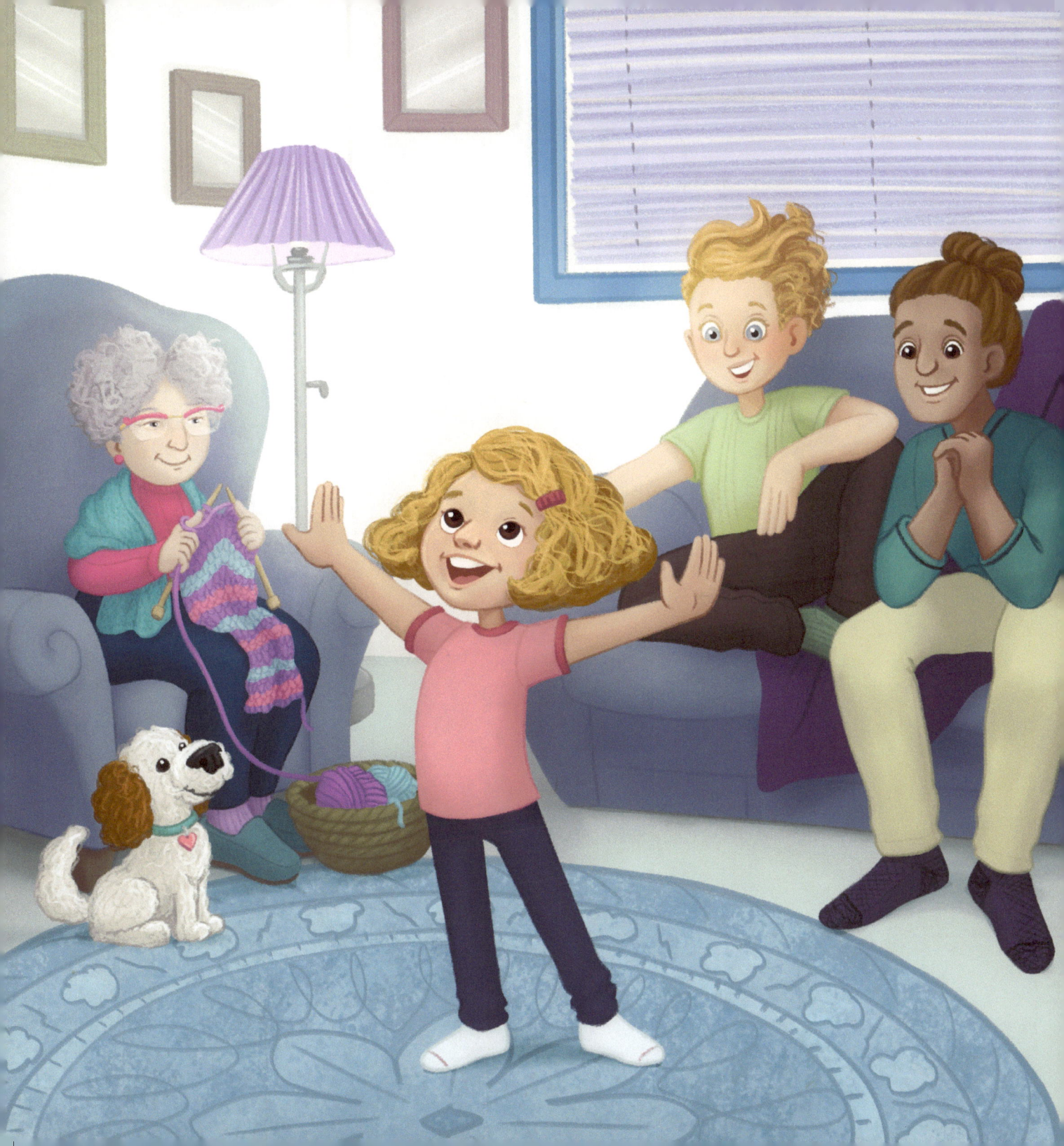

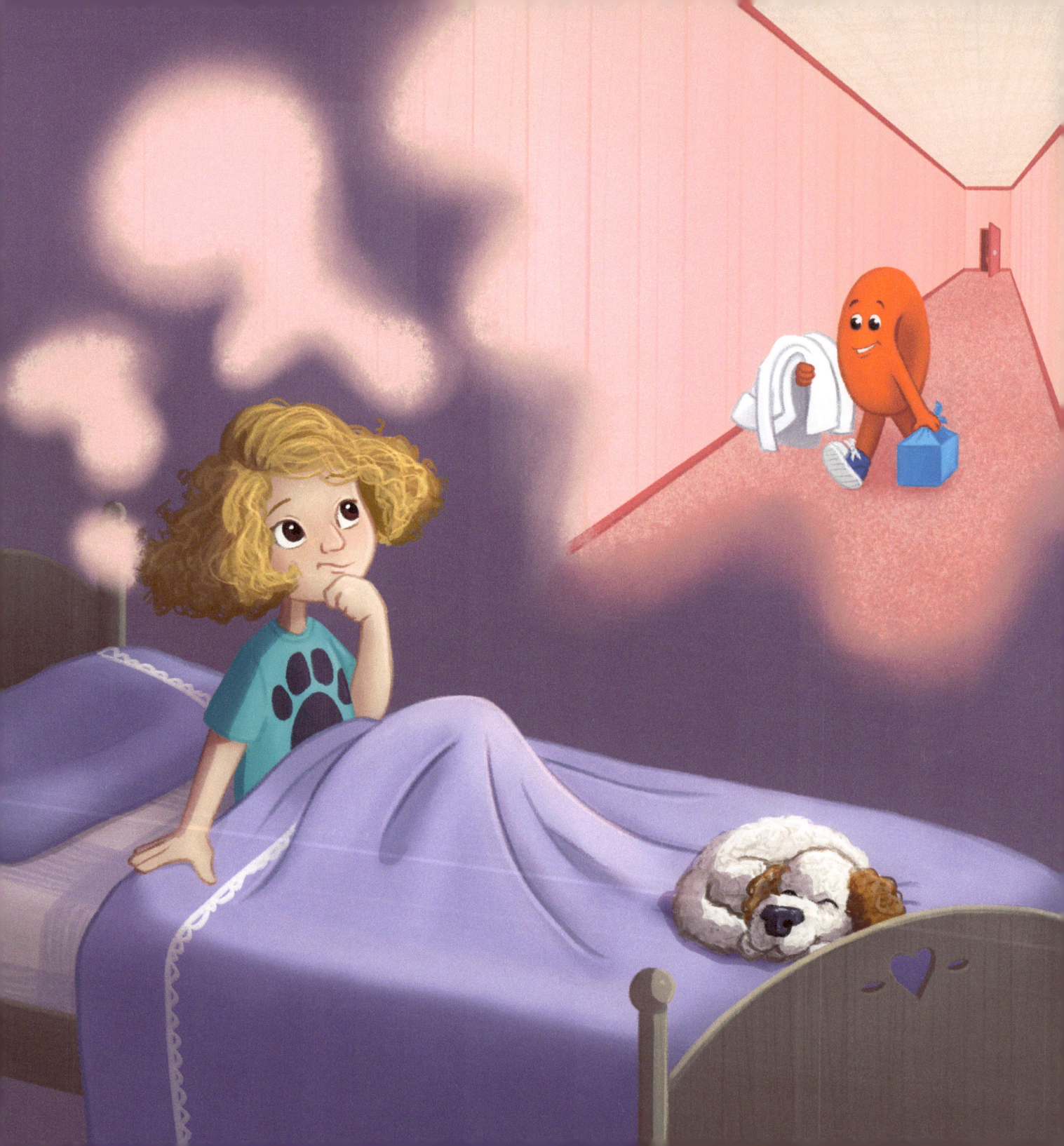

After an exciting day, Charlie is tucked under her cozy blanket in bed, her dog snoozing peacefully at her feet. She can't stop thinking about her **heart**. Her big, curious eyes stare at the ceiling as she thinks about how blood moves through the **heart's chambers**. What does it look like inside?

As her eyes grow heavy, and her bedroom starts to change, she began to drift into a dream. The walls shimmer and swirl, becoming soft and hazy, like clouds painted with her imagination. In her dream, something magical appears—Mr. Red!

Mr. Red is a cheerful **red blood cell**, round and bright. He has big, kind eyes, a wide, welcoming smile, and tiny hands that hold a white lab coat and a little blue box.

Charlie tilts her head in amazement. "Who ... who are you?" she whispers.

"I'm Mr. Red, and I am here to show you how the **heart** works!" His voice is full of excitement. At that moment, Charlie notices a soft, rhythmic sound echoing in the air: ***lub-dub, lub-dub***. It feels steady and strong, like the **heartbeat** of a hidden adventure waiting to begin

"Hey there, Charlie!" chirps Mr. Red, with bright sneakers and a friendly smile. "I'm one of the many travelers in the **heart**, and I've got an important delivery to make! Right now, I'm carrying a special package I need to drop off, and I've got another waiting for me to pick up. Want to come along on my journey?"

Charlie's eyes light up. "I'd love to, Mr. Red! Can you tell me what package you need to pick up?"

"Of course!" Mr. Red replies. "Right now, I'm carrying a package full of waste called **carbon dioxide**. I'll deliver it to the **lungs**, where it will be sent out of your body when you exhale. After that, I'll pick up **oxygen**—our most important cargo—and carry it to its destination: the **brain**!"

Charlie grins, excited to join Mr. Red on his incredible adventure. "Let's go!" she says.

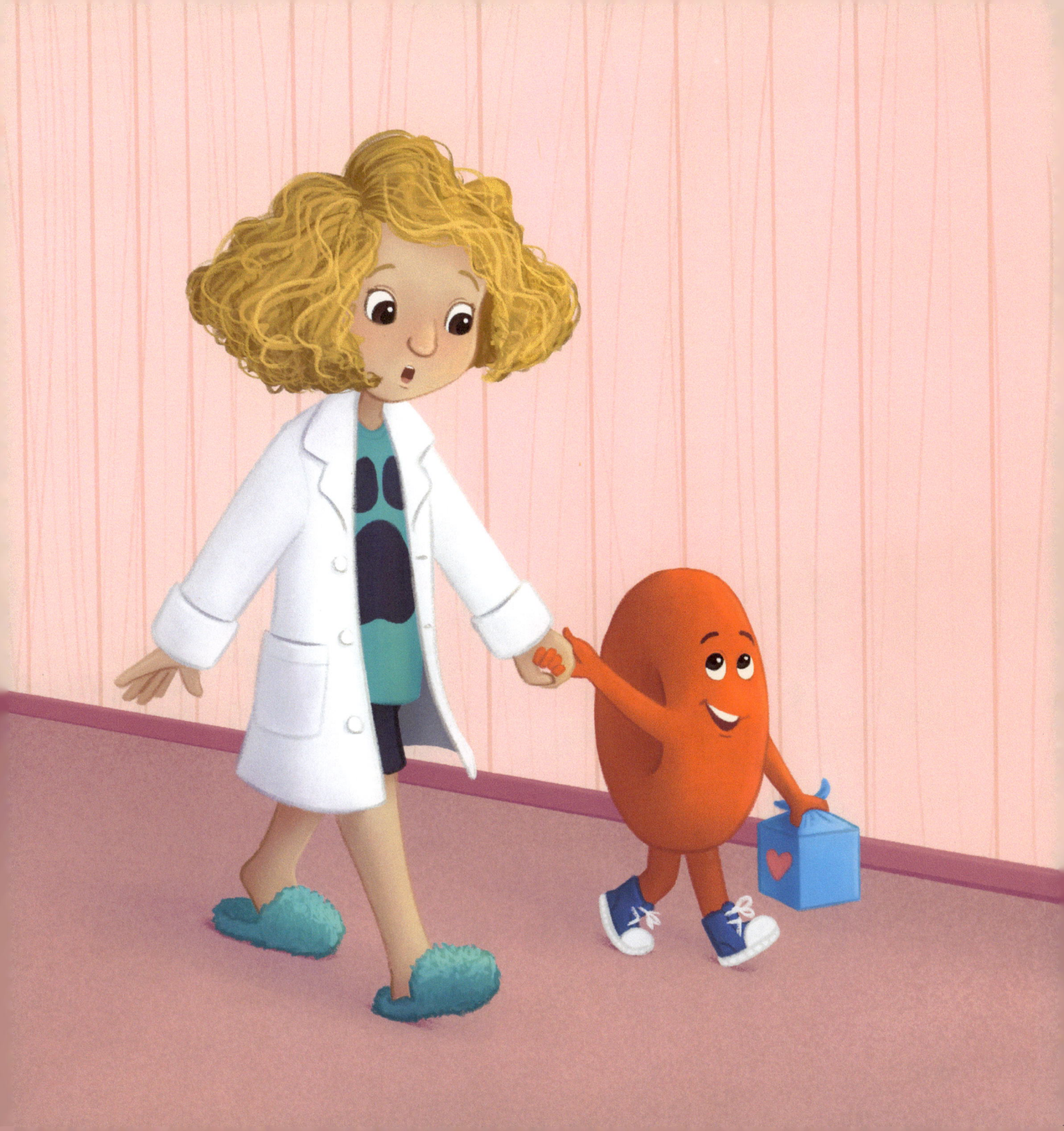

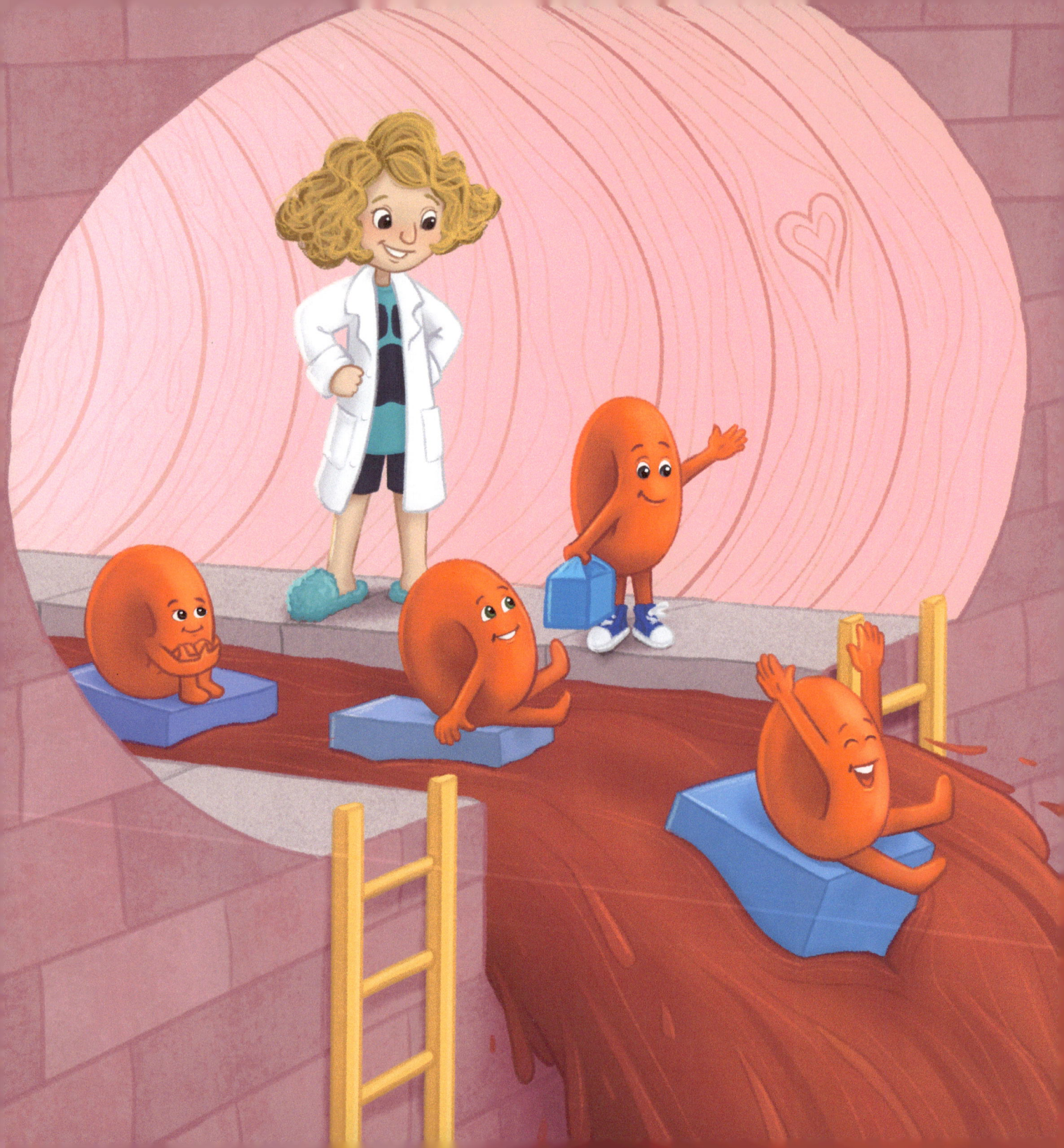

Mr. Red and Charlie are surrounded by other **red blood cells** zooming past on their important journeys. "Right now, we're in the **superior vena cava**," Mr. Red explains, gesturing to the large tunnel they're traveling through. "It's one of the main **blood vessels** that carries blood back to the **heart**. We'll be right inside the **heart** if we follow this path!"

"This is incredible!" Charlie says, her voice filled with awe. The tunnel is alive with movement—**red blood cells** riding currents of blood like adventurers on a river. She can't believe she's getting a close-up view of how her body works.

After sliding into the **heart**, Charlie and Mr. Red find themselves in a fascinating new space. "Welcome to the **right atrium**!" Mr. Red announces, waving his hand toward the room. "This is the first **chamber** of the **heart**. It's where most of the blood from the body gathers before continuing its journey."

Charlie looks around, and the room feels cozy, almost like a waiting room for the hardworking **red blood cells**. "It's smaller than I expected," but her eyes land on a grand set of intricate doors with swirling patterns that look like they are made of strong, flexible material. "What are those?" she asks, looking at the doors.

"Those are flaps, called the **tricuspid valve**," Mr. Red explains. "Think of them as the **heart's** one-way gates! They'll open to let us move into the next **chamber** while making sure blood doesn't flow backward. Pretty neat, right?"

Charlie nods, her curiosity growing. "Let's go through the gates and see where they lead!"

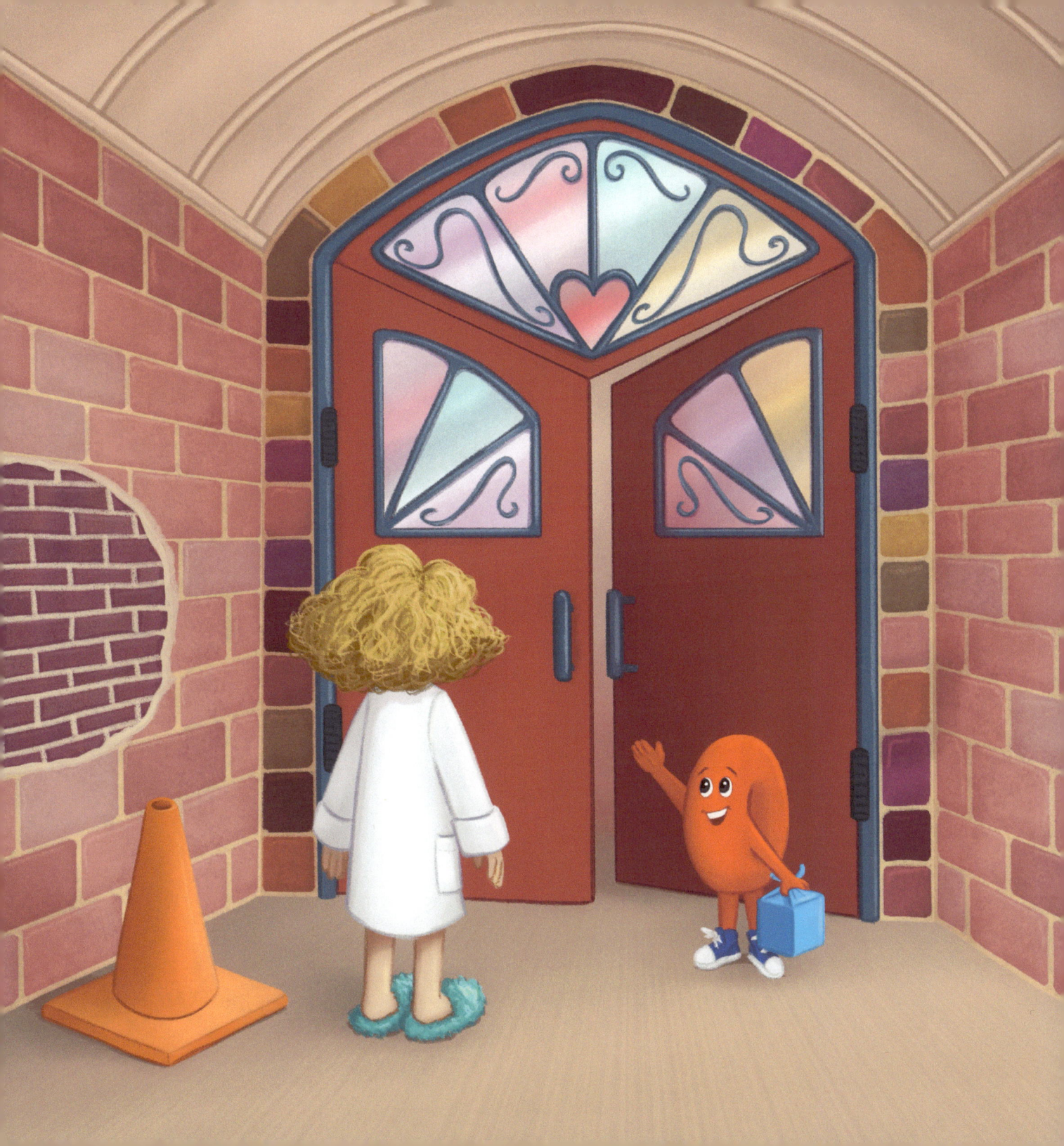

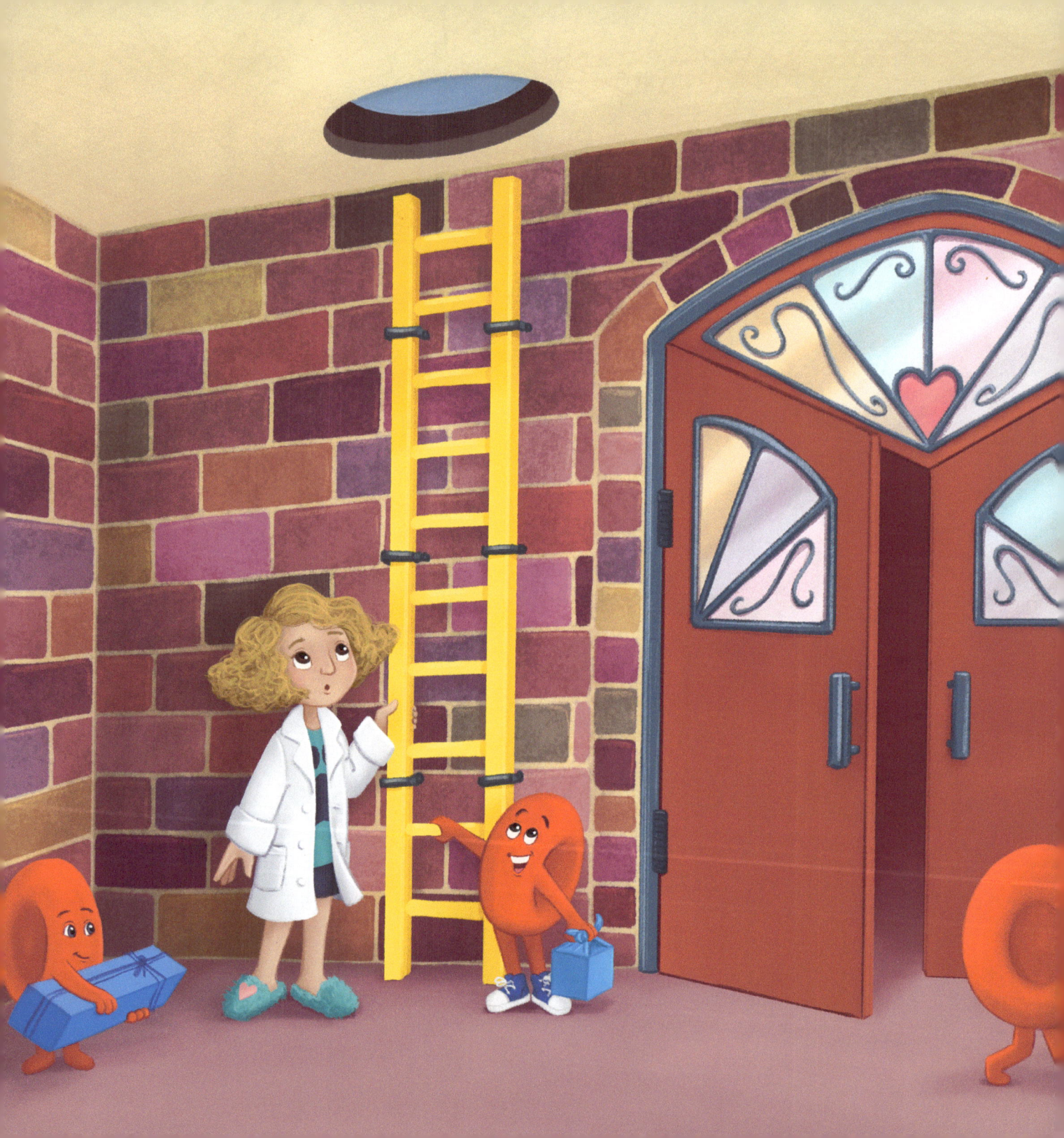

As Charlie and Mr. Red step into the next **chamber**, the **right ventricle**, Charlie immediately notices the walls. They look thick and strong. Curiously, she turns to ask, "Are we in a pumping **chamber**, Mr. Red?"

"That's exactly right, Charlie!" Mr. Red replies with a smile. "This is the **right ventricle**, one of the **heart's** powerful pumping **chambers**. After we leave this room, we'll travel through a special **vessel** called the **pulmonary trunk**, or **artery**. It's like a big tunnel that will take us to the **lungs**, where we'll pick up an important package—**oxygen**!"

"This is amazing! Let's keep going—I can't wait to see what's next!" Charlie exclaims.

As they make their way to the **lungs**, Charlie and Mr. Red find themselves in a hallway alive with motion, as packages are constantly crossing to each side. Charlie is in awe as she takes it all in. "This is incredible!" she says. "Do these **oxygen** and **carbon dioxide** packages move through this hallway all the time?"

"What a great question, Charlie!" Mr. Red replies, pausing to pick up his new package of **oxygen**. "Yes, they do! This process is called gas exchange. It's how **oxygen** enters our blood to reach our **cells** and how waste, like **carbon dioxide**, is removed."

Charlie watches the **red blood cells** move quickly and carefully. "Wow! It's like a super-efficient delivery system!" she exclaims.

Mr. Red grins. "That's exactly right! Now that we have our **oxygen** package, we must deliver it to the **brain**. But first, we must make a quick stop back at the **heart**, and this time, we travel through the oxygenated side!"

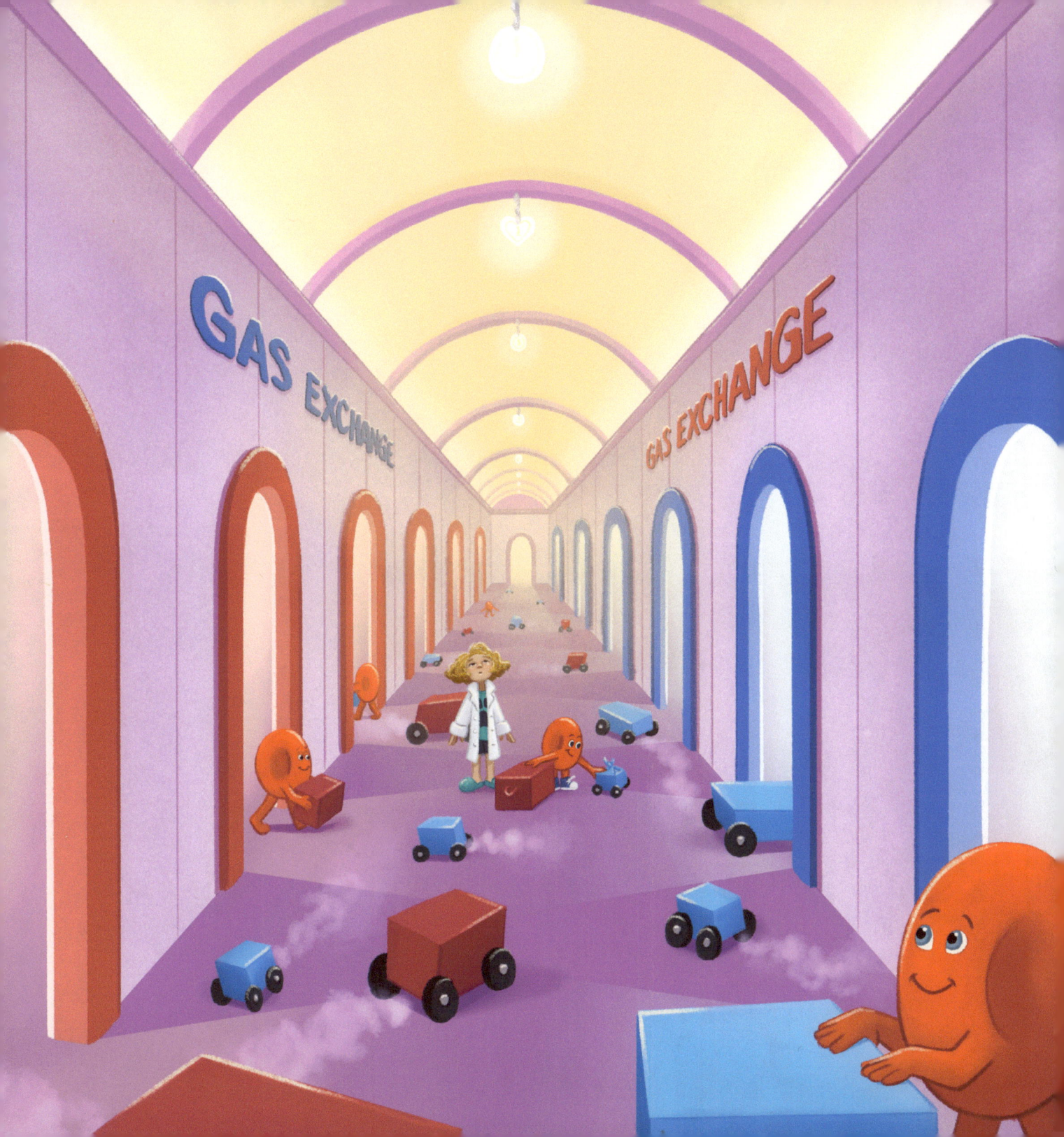

GAS EXCHANGE   GAS EXCHANGE

EXITING
PULMONARY
VEIN

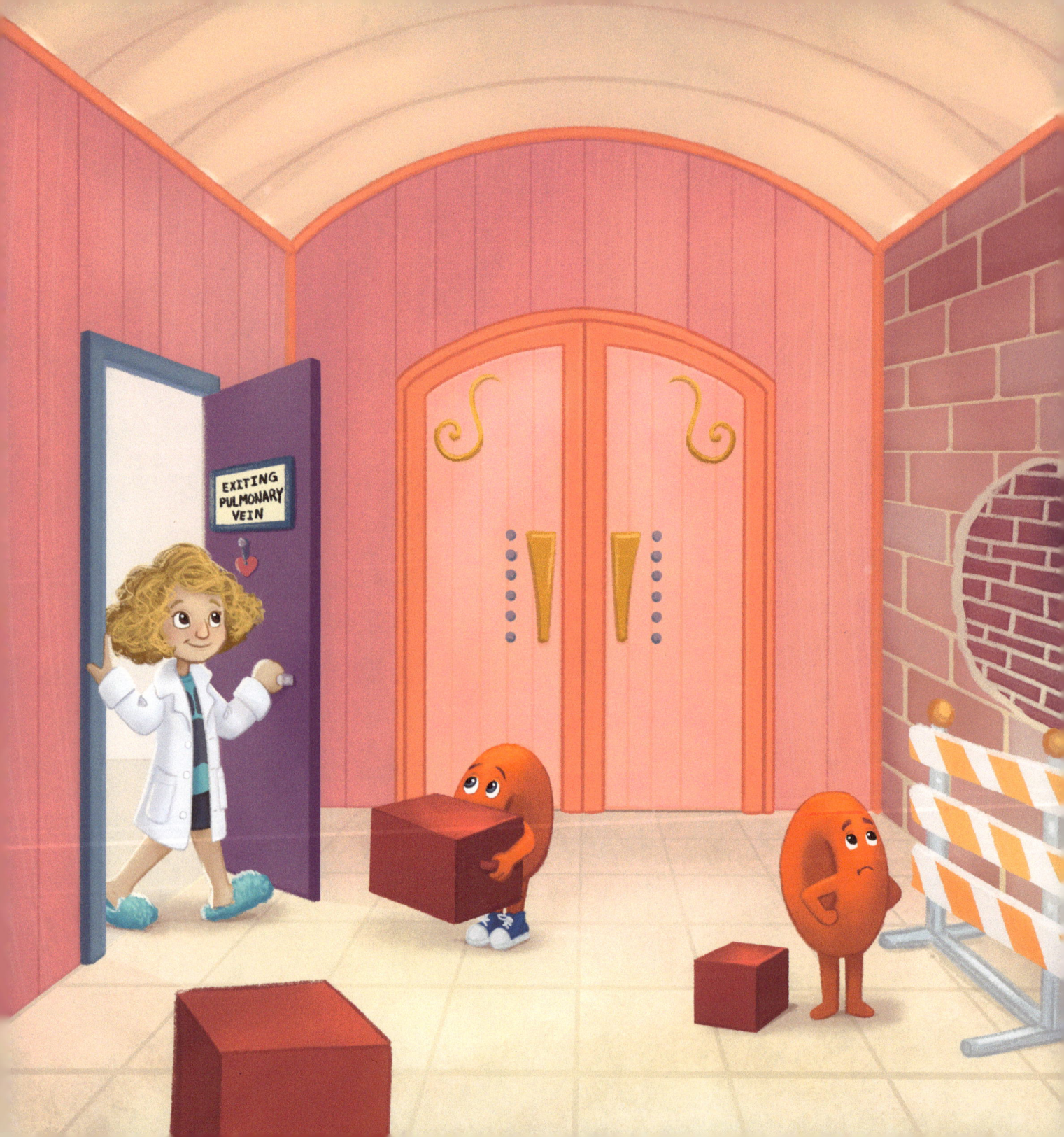

Mr. Red and Charlie enter a new receiving **chamber**, the **left atrium**. Mr. Red looks around proudly and says, "This room is special, Charlie, because it receives oxygen-rich blood. From here, the **oxygen** will travel to the entire body!"

Charlie sees the large double doors ahead and takes a deep breath. "So, the **left ventricle** is next after passing through this other valve?" she asks, realizing her adventure may be nearing its end.

Mr. Red nods. "That's right! This valve is called the **bicuspid valve**. Are you ready for the final step of our journey?"

Although sad that her adventure might be ending, Charlie feels excited to see how it all works. "I'm ready!" she says, her curiosity burning brightly.

Mr. Red pauses and gestures around the room after entering the **left ventricle**. "Take a look at this **chamber**, Charlie," he says. "Do you notice the walls are thicker than the last pumping **chamber**? That's because the **left ventricle** has the most important job—it needs to be strong enough to squeeze and push blood to the entire body!" Charlie nods, marveling at the **heart's** many functions.

"Well, Charlie, it's time to continue my journey alone. I'll travel through the **aorta**, the largest **blood vessel** in the body, to deliver this package to the **brain**. After that, I'll continue this cycle and keep going to other **organs**.

Charlie waves as Mr. Red exits toward the aorta. "I loved being your travel buddy, Mr. Red!" she calls out.

"And I loved having you as my partner, Charlie!" Mr. Red exclaims. "Keep learning and exploring—you've got a whole body full of adventures ahead of you!"

As Mr. Red disappears through the **aorta**, Charlie takes a deep breath and smiles, ready to share everything she's learned about the **heart** with her classmates

THIS WAY to the AORTA

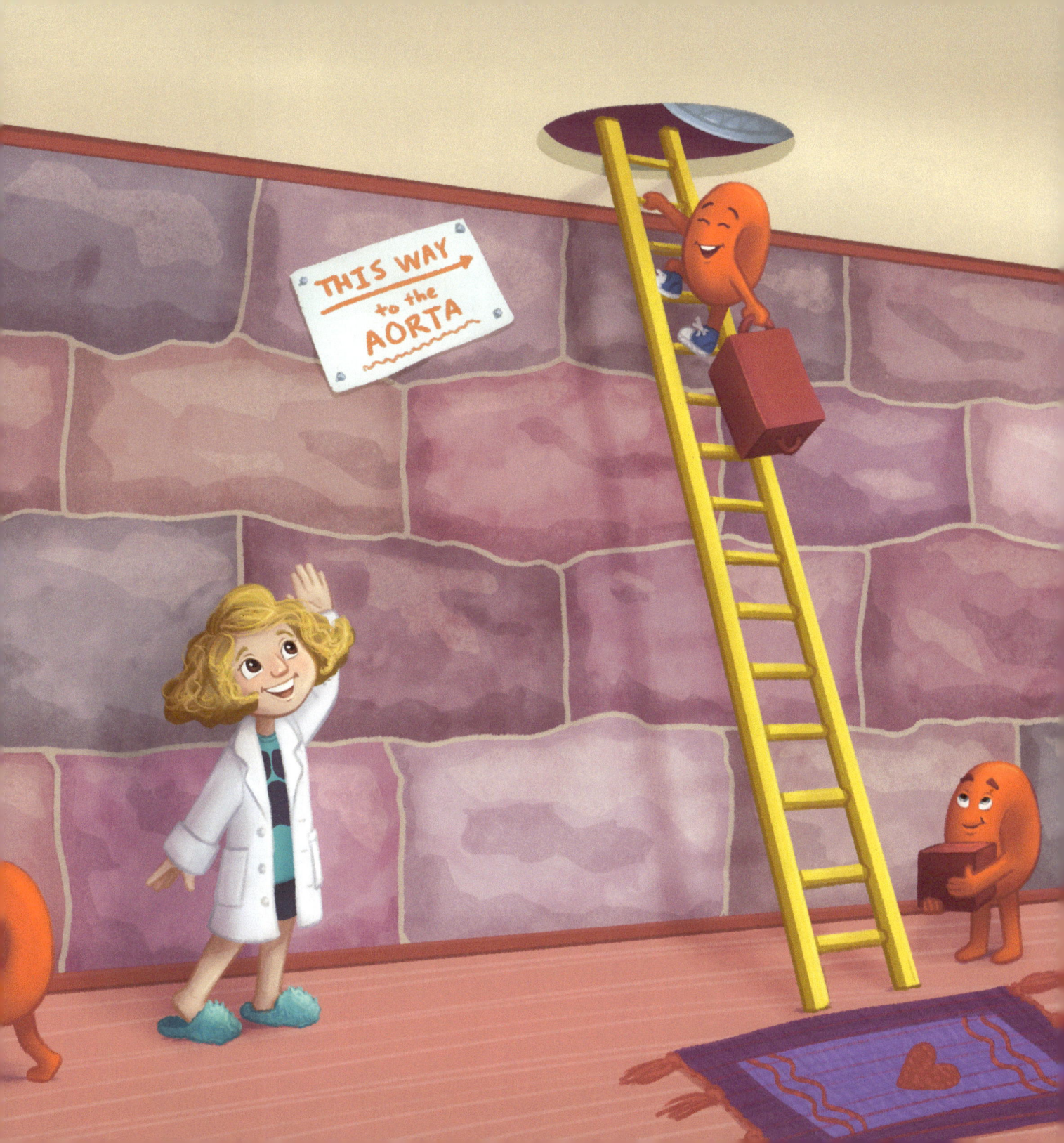

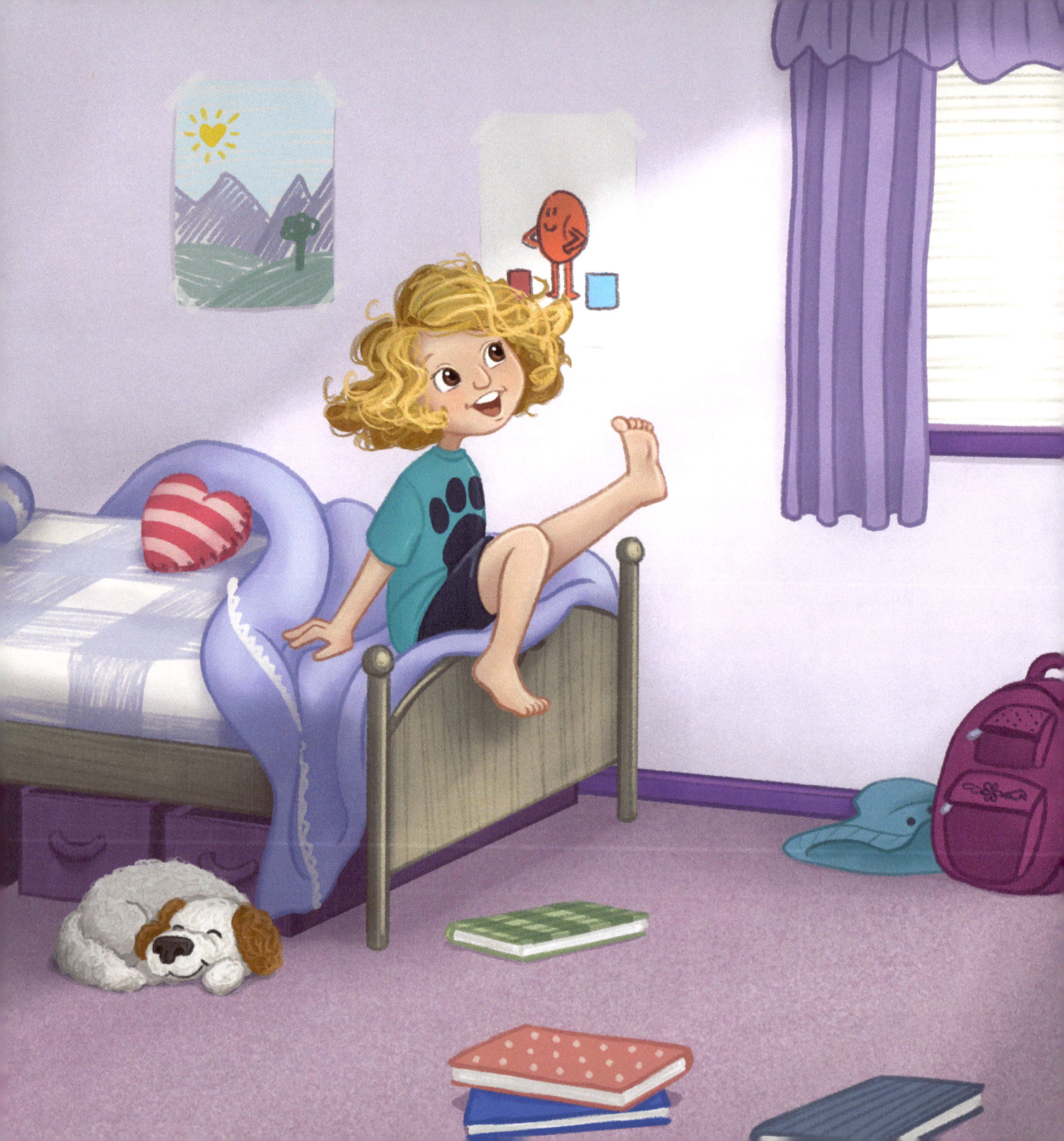

As sunlight streams through her window, Charlie stretches and sits up in bed with a big smile. She realizes that her incredible journey with Mr. Red was only a dream—but it felt so real!

Thanks to her adventure, Charlie is bursting with excitement and new knowledge about how the **heart** and blood work together to keep the body alive.

"I can't wait to tell everyone at school about my anatomical adventure!" she exclaims, hopping out of bed. With her **heart** full of curiosity, Charlie is ready to share her story and keep exploring the wonders of the human body.

Back at school, Charlie is overflowing with enthusiasm as she gathers her friends to share her fantastic dream. With her arms stretched wide and the need to share her recent adventure, she describes every detail she can remember.

Her friends listen while their eyes light up with curiosity. Charlie's energy is contagious, and soon, they're all eager to discover what adventures their science lessons will bring next.

"Our bodies are incredible!" she exclaims, practically bouncing. "The **heart** is just the beginning—there's so much more to explore! I can't wait to learn about the next human anatomy system!"

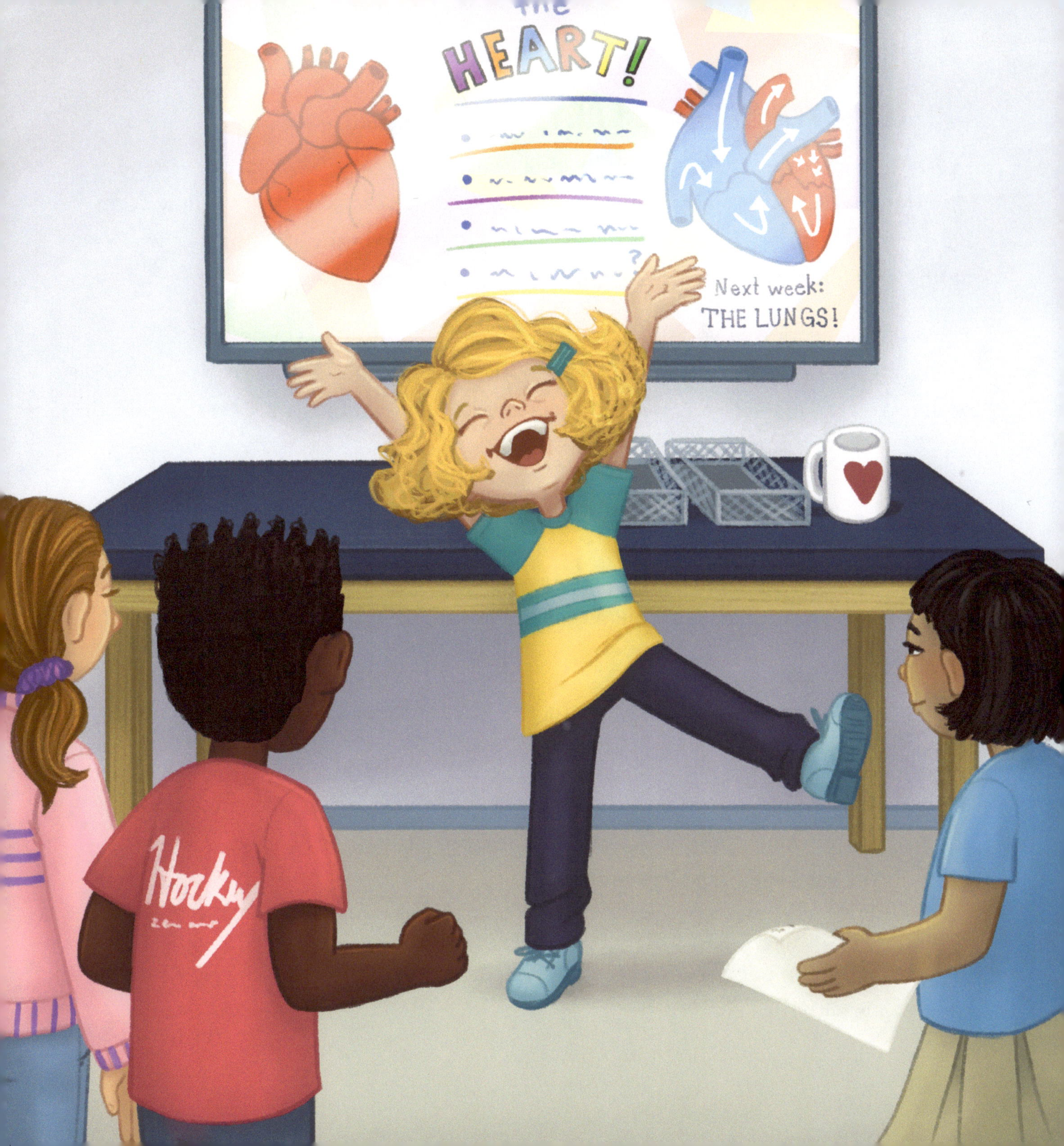
HEART!
Next week:
THE LUNGS!
Hockey

WELCOME TO THE GLOSSARY!

Learning the human body is like unlocking a whole new language! As you've read through **Charlie's Anatomical Adventure**, you've come across words that may seem big and tricky at first, but don't worry! Each bolded term in the story has a clear definition right here in the glossary to help you learn and remember.

Think of this section as your personal dictionary for anatomy—your guide to mastering the language of anatomy. The more you learn these terms, the better you'll understand the incredible systems that keep you healthy and strong. Happy learning!

Adipose: of or relating to fat

Aorta: the great arterial trunk that carries blood from the heart to be distributed by arteries through the body

Artery/Arteries: any of the tubular vessels that carry blood from the heart through the body

Atrium (left and right): a chamber of the heart that receives blood from the veins and forces it into a ventricle

Bicuspid valve: a structure (also known as the mitral valve) that closes temporarily and permits movement of fluid in one direction only; this specific valve is located between the left atrium and left ventricle only

Brain: the portion of the central nervous system that is the organ of thought and the central control point for the nervous system, is enclosed within the skull, and is continuous with the spinal cord

Carbon dioxide: a heavy colorless gas (CO2) that is formed especially by the burning and breaking down of organic substances (as in respiration)

Cardiologist: a physician who studies the heart and its action and diseases

Cells: one of the tiny units that are the basic building blocks of living things

Exercise: bodily activity for the sake of physical fitness

Heart: a hollow muscular organ that expands and contracts to move blood through the arteries, veins, and capillaries

Heartbeat: a single contracting and expanding of the heart

(Heart) Chambers: an enclosed space or compartment within the heart

Lub-Dub: the characteristic sounds of a normal heartbeat as heard when listening to heart sounds

Lungs: paired organs forming the special breathing structure of vertebrates that breathe air

Muscle: a body tissue that can contract and produce motion

Nutrient: a substance or ingredient that promotes growth, provides energy, and maintains life

Organ: a structure that consists of cells and tissues and is specialized to do a particular task

Oxygen: an element that is found in water, rocks, free as a colorless tasteless odorless gas, and is necessary for life

Pulmonary trunk: an artery that carries blood containing high amounts of carbon dioxide from the right side of the heart to the lungs

Red Blood Cell: a reddish cell of the blood that contains hemoglobin

Superior/Inferior vena cava: a blood vessel that returns blood to the heart from the upper or lower part of the body

Tricuspid valve: a structure that closes temporarily or permits movement of fluid in one direction only. This specific valve is located between the right atrium and right ventricle only

Vein/Veins: one of the blood vessels that carry blood back to the heart

Ventricle (left and right): a chamber of the heart which receives blood from an atrium and forces blood into an artery

Vessels (blood): any of the tubes through which blood circulates in the body

*Definitions listed originate from the Merriam-Webster.com Dictionary but may be slightly altered for a kid-friendly version.

HEART HUNT CHALLENGE!

Did you notice the hidden hearts throughout Charlie's adventure? Every page has at least one heart cleverly hidden in the illustrations—sometimes it's big and obvious, and other times it's small and sneaky!

HOW TO PLAY:

Start at the beginning: Go back to the beginning and look at the illustrations carefully.

Search for the hearts: Find at least one heart on every page. It could be part of the background, an object, or even a design!

Keep count: Write down the number of hearts you find on each page in a notebook or a piece of paper.

Compare with friends: See if you and your friends found the same hearts. Did anyone find extra hidden ones?

BONUS CHALLENGE:

Find all the unique hearts: Some hearts are in different shapes, colors, or patterns. Can you find them all?

Create your own scavenger hunt: Draw your favorite scene from the book and hide your hearts in the picture. Share it with family and friends to play!

Enjoy the hunt and remember—hearts are everywhere if you look closely!

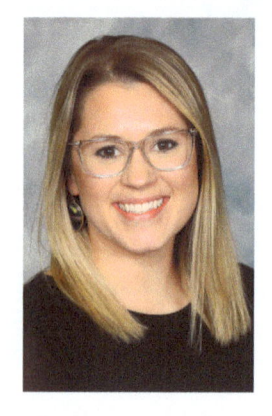

ABOUT THE AUTHOR

Abbey Breckling is an enthusiastic human anatomy educator and researcher and is passionate about making the wonders of the human body exciting for young minds. With a background in exercise physiology and anatomy, she brings her love of science to life in her children's book, designed to spark interest and wonder. Abbey's innovative approach incorporates elements of play and exploration, aiming to spark curiosity to make learning about anatomy fun and engaging. Through this book, she hopes to inspire the next generation of scientists and explorers. She invites young readers on an adventurous journey, encouraging them to discover the magic within themselves and the incredible world of anatomy.

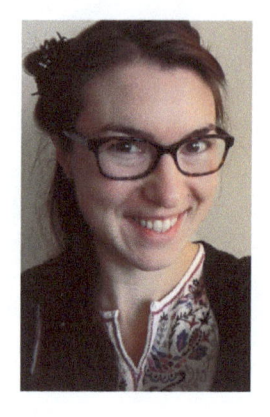

ABOUT THE ILLUSTRATOR

Melissa Lettis is an illustrator and a storyteller who loves bringing expressive, unique, and endearing characters to life. Growing up in Alaska, she developed a love of nature paired with a love of being cozy. She currently lives in Pennsylvania, where she illustrates, dances, drinks absurd amounts of tea, and befriends stories in their many forms.

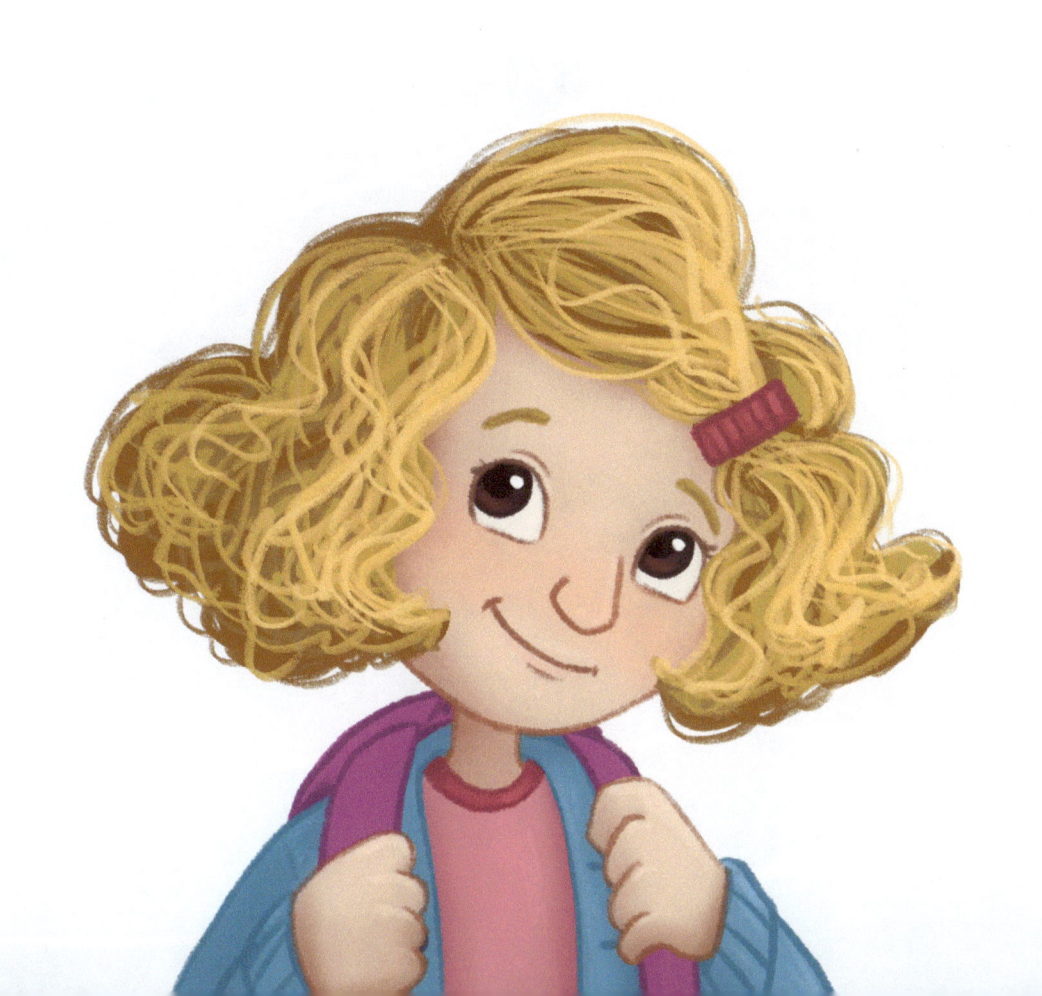

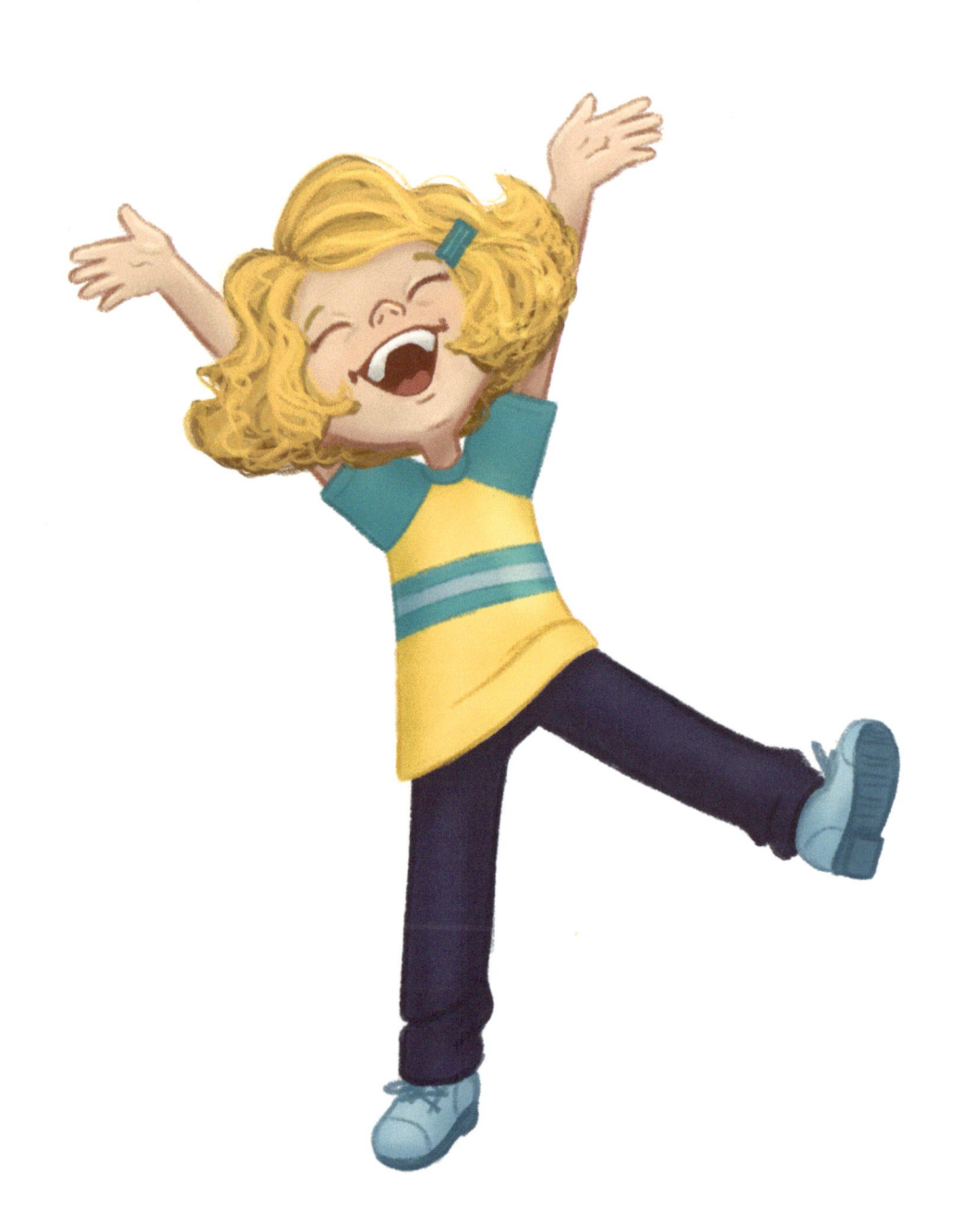

www.ingramcontent.com/pod-product-compliance
Lightning Source LLC
Jackson TN
JSHW040951310125
78003JS00013B/13